ENDOMORPH WEIGHT LOSS BLUEPRINT

SCIENCE-BASED STRATEGIES TO SHED POUNDS AND BOOST METABOLISM NATURALLY

TABLE OF CONTENTS

UNDERSTANDING THE ENDOMORPH BODY TYPE

In the realm of body types, the endomorph is often recognized by certain distinguishing physical characteristics: a softer, rounder physique, a tendency to store fat more easily, and generally shorter limbs compared to other body types. Originating from the somatotype theory developed by Dr. William Sheldon in the 1940s, the endomorph body type is one of three primary classifications, alongside ectomorphs and mesomorphs. While this system is not a strict rule but rather a general framework, many people find that understanding these body types helps them tailor their approach to fitness and weight management more effectively.

Endomorphs generally possess a slower metabolic rate, meaning they may not burn calories as quickly as other body types. This characteristic often results in easier weight gain and increased fat storage, particularly in areas like the hips, thighs, and abdomen. These metabolic differences are due to a combination of genetics and individual biology.

Because of this, endomorphs tend to respond differently to common weight loss strategies and may require unique approaches to achieve sustainable results.

Beyond physical traits, the endomorph body type also affects hormonal and metabolic responses, particularly when it comes to carbohydrate processing. Endomorphs often exhibit a higher degree of insulin sensitivity, meaning they are more prone to store carbohydrates as fat rather than using them for immediate energy. This predisposition can make conventional high-carb diets less effective and sometimes counterproductive for endomorphs, as excess carbs are more easily converted to fat stores.

However, while the endomorph body type presents challenges, it also comes with advantages. Endomorphs are often naturally strong and have a powerful lower body, which can be an asset in strength training and physical activities requiring endurance. Embracing these strengths and recognizing areas where the endomorph body type might benefit from specific strategies are key to a balanced and effective approach to health.

HOW THIS BLUEPRINT WILL HELP YOU ACHIEVE YOUR GOALS

The *Endomorph Weight Loss Blueprint* is designed to provide practical, science-based strategies tailored to the needs of endomorphs who want to lose weight, build lean muscle, and improve their overall health. This book is not a one-size-fits-all solution but rather a guide that considers the unique physiology of endomorphs to help them work with their bodies, not against them. Whether you're aiming to shed a few pounds, tone your physique, or adopt a healthier lifestyle, this blueprint offers the tools, insights, and actionable steps you need to reach your goals.

Throughout this book, we'll delve into key topics such as nutrition, exercise, metabolism, and mental health, all designed with the endomorph body type in mind. Each chapter will build upon the last, guiding you step-by-step through a sustainable weight loss journey. From understanding how macronutrients affect your body to choosing the right types of exercise, this blueprint offers a holistic approach that goes beyond traditional diet and exercise plans. You'll gain the knowledge needed to make informed choices about your health, and learn how to adjust your lifestyle in a way that's manageable and enjoyable.

One of the primary focuses of this blueprint is achieving sustainable results. While quick-fix diets and intense workout regimens may yield rapid results, they're often difficult to maintain in the long run. For endomorphs, adopting a consistent, gradual approach to weight loss is typically more effective and manageable. This guide encourages consistency over intensity, helping you establish habits that align with your lifestyle rather than disrupting it. You'll learn to develop a mindset that supports lasting change, which is crucial for overcoming obstacles and staying motivated on your journey.

Additionally, this blueprint takes a science-based approach to address common challenges and setbacks that endomorphs face. You'll find practical advice grounded in research and real-world experience, so you can navigate common pitfalls like plateaus, emotional eating, and the struggle to stay motivated. By the end of this book, you'll have a personalized strategy that empowers you to make meaningful changes while celebrating the unique strengths of your body type.

A BALANCED APPROACH TO WEIGHT LOSS

When it comes to weight loss, many people gravitate toward extreme approaches: restrictive diets, grueling workouts, or drastic lifestyle changes. However, for endomorphs, a balanced approach to weight loss often proves to be the most effective and sustainable. This blueprint emphasizes balance in three key areas: nutrition, exercise, and mindset. By finding harmony between these aspects, endomorphs can achieve their weight loss goals while maintaining physical, mental, and emotional well-being.

Balanced Nutrition: The cornerstone of weight loss for endomorphs is adopting a nutrition plan that respects their unique metabolic needs. Because endomorphs are more sensitive to insulin and store carbohydrates as fat more readily, they often benefit from a lower-carb, higher-protein diet that stabilizes blood sugar levels and reduces cravings. However, this does not mean that endomorphs should avoid carbohydrates altogether. Instead, the focus should be on high-quality, complex carbohydrates—such as vegetables, whole grains, and legumes—that provide sustained energy and prevent rapid spikes in blood sugar.

Protein is particularly important for endomorphs, as it supports muscle maintenance, which in turn boosts metabolic rate. This book offers guidance on portion sizes, food choices, and meal timing to help endomorphs achieve a balanced, nutritious diet without feeling deprived. The goal is not to restrict but to empower you to make healthier choices that work in your favor.

Effective Exercise: Exercise is another essential component of a balanced weight loss strategy, and for endomorphs, the type of exercise matters greatly. While cardio exercises are effective for burning calories, they alone may not provide the muscle-building benefits that endomorphs need to boost their metabolism. Strength training is particularly beneficial, as it builds lean muscle mass, which increases the body's calorie-burning potential even at rest. High-intensity interval training (HIIT) can also be effective, as it provides both cardio and strength benefits in a short amount of time.

The exercise routines provided in this book are designed to be adaptable and enjoyable, allowing you to build strength, improve endurance, and support weight loss without overloading yourself. Consistency is prioritized over intensity, making it easier to integrate exercise into your daily life.

Mindset and Motivation: Finally, mindset is a crucial component of sustainable weight loss. The journey to health is as much mental as it is physical, and endomorphs often face unique psychological challenges. Frustration over slower results or perceived setbacks can lead to discouragement and emotional eating. This blueprint encourages a compassionate, patient mindset that focuses on progress rather than perfection.

Through mindfulness techniques, self-reflection exercises, and goal-setting strategies, you'll learn to reframe setbacks as learning opportunities rather than failures. Developing a resilient mindset is essential for maintaining consistency, even when results take time. By focusing on sustainable progress, you'll build a foundation for lifelong health and fitness.

CHAPTER 1

THE ENDOMORPH BODY TYPE: TRAITS AND
CHALLENGES

1.1 CHARACTERISTICS OF AN ENDOMORPH

The endomorph body type is one of the three somatotypes, or natural body types, identified in somatotype theory. Endomorphs tend to have a larger frame, higher body fat percentage, and are often characterized by a rounded body shape, particularly around the hips, thighs, and midsection. People with endomorphic traits commonly have softer, wider bodies with shorter limbs, often making them more stocky or curvaceous compared to other body types. Unlike ectomorphs, who are naturally lean, or mesomorphs, who are naturally muscular, endomorphs are predisposed to store fat more easily.

This body type can impact various aspects of a person's physiology, such as metabolism and fat distribution, due to their slower metabolic rates. Additionally, endomorphs often experience greater difficulty building muscle mass while simultaneously losing fat, as their bodies are more efficient at storing calories. However, it's important to note that while endomorphs may have a genetic predisposition to a certain body structure, lifestyle factors—including diet, exercise, and stress management—play a substantial role in determining their overall health and physique.

Due to their higher body fat levels and larger frame, endomorphs may possess significant strength, even if it's not immediately visible. This strength gives endomorphs a powerful advantage in certain physical activities, such as powerlifting, where lower-body strength and a sturdy frame can provide enhanced performance. With the right approach to fitness and nutrition, endomorphs can develop a leaner, stronger body while working within their genetic potential. Recognizing the unique characteristics of their body type empowers endomorphs to better understand their physical needs and embrace a sustainable approach to fitness.

1.2 WHY ENDOMORPHS GAIN WEIGHT EASILY

Endomorphs have a naturally slower metabolism than ectomorphs or mesomorphs, making it more challenging for them to burn calories at the same rate. Several factors contribute to this slower metabolic rate. First, endomorphs tend to have lower muscle mass, which directly influences the basal metabolic rate (BMR), or the number of calories the body needs to function at rest. Muscle tissue is metabolically active, meaning it burns more calories even when the body is inactive. Because endomorphs typically have less muscle mass, they may require fewer calories daily, making it easier to gain weight if caloric intake is not carefully managed.

Endomorphs are also often more insulin-sensitive, meaning their bodies respond strongly to the insulin hormone, which regulates blood sugar and energy storage. While insulin sensitivity has some benefits, such as efficient energy storage, it also makes endomorphs more prone to store excess carbohydrates as fat. For instance, when an endomorph consumes carbohydrates, their body may store this energy more readily in fat cells rather than using it for immediate energy. This means that endomorphs need to be more conscious of carbohydrate intake to avoid spikes in blood sugar that could lead to weight gain.

Furthermore, endomorphs tend to have a higher percentage of body fat, which may increase levels of the hormone leptin. Although leptin typically helps regulate hunger and energy balance, in some cases, higher body fat can lead to leptin resistance, where the brain doesn't receive accurate hunger signals. As a result, endomorphs might feel hungrier more often, leading to a cycle of overeating and weight gain. This, coupled with a lower resting metabolic rate, creates a challenging environment for endomorphs aiming to lose or maintain weight. It's essential for endomorphs to understand these biological predispositions so they can adopt tailored dietary strategies—such as reducing carbohydrate intake and prioritizing protein and healthy fats—to manage weight effectively.

1.3 COMMON MYTHS ABOUT ENDOMORPHS AND WEIGHT LOSS

Many misconceptions surround the endomorph body type, often leading to discouragement and frustration among those with endomorphic traits. One common myth is that endomorphs cannot lose weight, regardless of how hard they try. While it's true that endomorphs may face more obstacles due to their natural physiology, weight loss is not impossible. With a personalized approach that takes into account their unique metabolic needs, endomorphs can effectively lose weight and achieve a healthier body composition. Consistency in both diet and exercise, along with patience, is key to overcoming these challenges.

Another pervasive myth is that all endomorphs are "doomed" to have high body fat for life. This oversimplifies the complex relationship between genetics and lifestyle. Although genetics play a role in body composition, they do not determine the outcome. By implementing the right fitness strategies, endomorphs can reduce body fat and increase lean muscle mass, transforming their physique. Lifestyle adjustments, such as adopting a diet rich in lean proteins, healthy fats, and fiber, alongside regular exercise, can make a significant difference over time.

A third myth suggests that cardio alone is the solution for endomorphs who want to lose weight. However, while cardio exercises can aid in calorie burn and cardiovascular health, they are not the only—or even the most effective—strategy for endomorphs looking to lose fat. Strength training is particularly beneficial for endomorphs because it increases muscle mass, which, in turn, elevates their resting metabolic rate. By building more muscle, endomorphs can naturally burn more calories throughout the day, making it easier to manage their weight. Incorporating a balanced mix of cardio and strength training, as well as high-intensity interval training (HIIT), can yield optimal results for fat loss and muscle gain.

Finally, there is a common misconception that endomorphs should avoid eating carbohydrates altogether. While it's true that endomorphs may benefit from a controlled carbohydrate intake, avoiding carbohydrates entirely is neither necessary nor sustainable. Carbohydrates are an essential macronutrient and provide energy for workouts and daily activities. The key is to choose complex carbohydrates, such as whole grains, vegetables, and legumes, which release energy more slowly and help maintain stable blood sugar levels. These types of carbohydrates support sustained energy and are less likely to lead to fat storage compared to simple carbohydrates. For endomorphs, the focus should be on carbohydrate quality and portion control rather than total elimination.

CHAPTER 2

METABOLISM AND ENDOMORPHS

2.1 UNDERSTANDING METABOLISM: THE SCIENCE BEHIND IT

Metabolism is a complex, essential process through which our bodies convert the food and drink we consume into energy. It involves a series of chemical reactions that allow the body to grow, repair cells, and maintain essential functions such as breathing, digestion, and temperature regulation. Understanding metabolism's intricacies can help people, especially those with an endomorph body type, tailor their approach to diet, exercise, and overall lifestyle to better support weight loss and wellness goals.

At its core, metabolism can be broken down into two main categories: catabolism and anabolism. Catabolism is the process through which the body breaks down nutrients (like carbohydrates, fats, and proteins) to release energy. Anabolism, on the other hand, is the process of building and storing—constructing new cells, maintaining muscle, and storing fat as a backup source of energy. Metabolism is in a constant state of balancing these processes, depending on the body's needs at any given moment.

The rate at which these metabolic processes occur varies widely among individuals, and it's largely influenced by genetic factors, body composition, and lifestyle choices. For endomorphs, who often have a slower metabolic rate than other body types, the body tends to favor energy storage over burning calories. This predisposition can make weight management more challenging, as the body naturally leans toward retaining energy in the form of fat rather than quickly expending it.

It's important to note that metabolism isn't only active when you're engaged in physical activity. Even when at rest, your body continues to use energy for essential functions, known as the Basal Metabolic Rate (BMR). BMR accounts for a significant portion of daily calorie expenditure and is influenced by muscle mass, age, gender, and genetics. Understanding the science behind metabolism—and specifically how it differs for endomorphs—can empower individuals to work with their natural body chemistry to optimize weight loss and overall health.

2.2 METABOLIC RATE AND FAT STORAGE

One of the key challenges for endomorphs is their lower metabolic rate, which means they generally burn fewer calories at rest compared to other body types, such as ectomorphs or mesomorphs. This lower resting metabolic rate (RMR) is partly due to having less muscle mass, which is more metabolically active than fat tissue. Since muscle tissue burns more calories even when the body is at rest, individuals with a higher muscle-to-fat ratio have an easier time maintaining a faster metabolism. For endomorphs, building muscle can significantly impact their metabolic rate and can help offset some of the natural tendency toward fat storage.

When it comes to fat storage, the body's response to calorie intake and hormonal signals is essential to understand. For endomorphs, the body is more prone to store excess calories as fat, particularly when those calories come from carbohydrates. This tendency toward fat storage is linked to insulin sensitivity. Insulin is a hormone that helps regulate blood sugar levels by signaling cells to absorb glucose. While insulin sensitivity can be beneficial, as it allows cells to effectively utilize glucose, it can also contribute to fat storage when excess calories are consumed, particularly from refined or high-glycemic carbohydrates.

The body stores excess energy in fat cells, which can expand to accommodate additional fat deposits. For endomorphs, the body may be more efficient at this storage process, meaning that it's easier for them to gain weight and more challenging to lose it. This doesn't mean, however, that endomorphs are doomed to retain fat indefinitely. By understanding how their metabolism works and tailoring their diet and exercise plans accordingly, endomorphs can work toward maintaining a balanced energy intake and expenditure.

One effective strategy is to focus on reducing carbohydrate intake and emphasizing protein and healthy fats. Protein has a thermic effect, meaning it requires more energy to digest and process, which can give metabolism a temporary boost after eating. Additionally, lean muscle mass, supported by protein-rich diets and regular strength training, can help endomorphs increase their resting metabolic rate, making fat storage less likely and promoting lean muscle maintenance.

2.3 FACTORS AFFECTING YOUR METABOLISM

Several factors influence metabolic rate, and many of these are unique to each individual, particularly when it comes to body types. For endomorphs, knowing which factors they can control—and which are largely set by genetics—can help them make informed choices to support a faster metabolism.

1. Muscle Mass- Muscle tissue is metabolically active and burns more calories than fat tissue, even while the body is at rest. This is why strength training is particularly beneficial for endomorphs. By increasing lean muscle mass, endomorphs can enhance their resting metabolic rate and make it easier to maintain a healthy weight. Resistance exercises, such as weight lifting, bodyweight exercises, and high-intensity interval training (HIIT), are excellent ways to build muscle and stimulate the metabolism.

2. Hormones- Hormones play a significant role in metabolic processes and fat storage. For endomorphs, insulin sensitivity is a notable factor that can affect how the body processes carbohydrates. Additionally, hormones such as leptin and ghrelin, which regulate hunger and satiety, can impact eating patterns and, consequently, weight management. Ensuring stable blood sugar levels through balanced meals can help regulate hunger hormones and reduce overeating.

3. Age- Metabolism naturally slows down as people age, largely due to decreases in muscle mass and changes in hormone levels. For endomorphs, this means that it's especially important to focus on muscle-preserving activities as they age. Strength training, proper protein intake, and regular physical activity are all crucial for slowing age-related metabolic decline and maintaining a healthier body composition.

4. Physical Activity- While resting metabolic rate plays a significant role in overall energy expenditure, physical activity also has a profound impact. Exercise, particularly high-intensity and resistance training, can temporarily boost metabolism by causing the body to use more oxygen even after the workout is complete—a phenomenon known as excess post-exercise oxygen consumption (EPOC). By incorporating consistent physical activity into their routine, endomorphs can benefit from the metabolic boost and enhanced calorie burn associated with exercise.

5. Diet and Macronutrient Composition- The types of foods consumed can influence metabolism, as certain nutrients require more energy to process. Protein, for example, has a high thermic effect, which means the body uses more calories to digest it compared to carbohydrates or fats. For endomorphs, a diet higher in protein and lower in refined carbohydrates can help stabilize blood sugar levels, enhance satiety, and support muscle mass, all of which can positively impact metabolism. Eating smaller, balanced meals throughout the day may also help prevent blood sugar spikes, helping to manage insulin levels and reduce fat storage.

6. Hydration- Adequate hydration is essential for metabolic function, as water is involved in nearly all bodily processes, including the breakdown and transport of nutrients. Dehydration can slow metabolism, making it harder for endomorphs to burn calories efficiently. Drinking enough water throughout the day can help support metabolic function and improve overall energy expenditure.

7. Sleep- Quality sleep is critical for metabolic health. Poor sleep or lack of rest can disrupt hormone levels, particularly those related to hunger and satiety (leptin and ghrelin). For endomorphs, poor sleep may lead to increased appetite and a tendency to store more fat. Prioritizing good sleep hygiene, such as maintaining a consistent sleep schedule and creating a relaxing nighttime routine, can support both metabolism and weight management.

CHAPTER 3

NUTRITION ESSENTIALS FOR ENDOMORPHS

3.1 MACROS AND MICRONUTRIENTS EXPLAINED

Nutrition is the foundation of any health journey, especially for endomorphs who may need to take a more tailored approach to their diet to manage weight effectively. One of the primary components of any nutritional plan is understanding macronutrients (macros) and micronutrients and how they impact the body.

Macronutrients are nutrients that the body requires in larger quantities. They provide calories and are used for energy, growth, and maintenance. There are three main macronutrients:

- **Carbohydrates**: These are the body's primary source of energy. Carbohydrates are broken down into glucose, which fuels our muscles, brain, and other tissues. For endomorphs, however, excess carbohydrates—especially refined or high-glycemic ones—can lead to increased fat storage due to heightened insulin sensitivity. This doesn't mean endomorphs should eliminate carbs, but choosing the right kinds, like whole grains, vegetables, and legumes, can make a significant difference.

- **Proteins**: Proteins are essential for muscle maintenance and repair. For endomorphs, protein is particularly valuable because it not only supports lean muscle mass but also has a high thermic effect. This means the body burns more calories digesting protein compared to carbs or fats. Protein helps stabilize blood sugar levels, keeps you full for longer, and aids in reducing cravings. Good protein sources include lean meats, fish, eggs, beans, and plant-based options like tofu and tempeh.

- **Fats**: Though they have the highest calorie density of the macros, healthy fats are essential for brain function, hormone production, and nutrient absorption. Fats can also help endomorphs feel fuller longer, which may reduce overeating. Healthy fats, like those found in avocados, nuts, seeds, and olive oil, are preferable to saturated and trans fats. Including a moderate amount of healthy fats can support sustained energy levels and satiety.

Micronutrients—vitamins and minerals—are needed in smaller amounts but are vital for overall health. They help support immune function, cell production, and energy metabolism. For endomorphs, prioritizing foods rich in micronutrients can support healthy metabolic function and reduce inflammation, which is sometimes higher in those with a tendency toward weight gain.

Some key micronutrients for endomorphs include:

- **Vitamin D**: Helps with calcium absorption, supports immune health, and can improve mood and energy. Low vitamin D is sometimes linked to weight gain, so ensuring adequate intake, through sunlight exposure or foods like fatty fish, eggs, and fortified dairy products, is beneficial.
- **Magnesium**: Important for energy production, muscle function, and blood sugar regulation. Magnesium can be found in leafy greens, nuts, seeds, and whole grains.
- **B Vitamins**: Essential for energy production and metabolism. B vitamins are commonly found in leafy greens, eggs, and lean meats.

A balanced diet that prioritizes whole foods, lean proteins, healthy fats, and low-glycemic carbs, with an emphasis on micronutrient-rich options, can help endomorphs improve energy levels, metabolism, and overall well-being.

3.2 THE IDEAL DIET FOR ENDOMORPHS

The ideal diet for an endomorph should focus on stabilizing blood sugar, promoting satiety, and minimizing unnecessary calorie intake. Unlike fad diets or extreme restrictions, the endomorph-friendly diet emphasizes balance, sustainability, and personalization.

1. Prioritize Protein: For endomorphs, a diet high in protein can be particularly effective. Protein not only supports muscle retention but also has a thermogenic effect, meaning the body uses more energy to digest it. Including a good source of protein in each meal—such as chicken, fish, eggs, or plant-based options—can help stabilize blood sugar and reduce cravings.

2. Choose Low-Glycemic Carbohydrates: Carbohydrates are not the enemy, but the type of carbs consumed makes a big difference. Low-glycemic, high-fiber carbs are digested more slowly, resulting in gradual blood sugar increases rather than sharp spikes. Foods like quinoa, sweet potatoes, lentils, and most vegetables provide steady energy without promoting fat storage. For endomorphs, limiting refined sugars, white flour, and processed snacks can help avoid rapid insulin spikes, which can lead to fat gain.

3. Incorporate Healthy Fats: Healthy fats can be an endomorph's ally in weight management. Fats slow digestion, leading to prolonged feelings of fullness, which can help prevent overeating. Omega-3 fatty acids, found in foods like salmon, chia seeds, and walnuts, have anti-inflammatory properties and support heart health, which is particularly beneficial for individuals with higher body fat. Including small amounts of fats like olive oil, nuts, and seeds in meals provides essential nutrients and helps regulate hunger.

4. Maintain Portion Control: While focusing on nutrient-dense foods is key, portion control also plays an essential role in maintaining a caloric balance. Endomorphs may benefit from slightly smaller meals spread throughout the day to keep metabolism steady and prevent overeating. Monitoring portion sizes of starchy carbs and fats, which can quickly add calories, can prevent unintentional weight gain. Smaller, balanced meals can also help regulate energy and support consistent metabolic function.

5. Plan for Consistency, Not Perfection: The endomorph-friendly diet is one that's sustainable and realistic. Building a pattern of balanced meals and mindful choices, rather than aiming for perfection, leads to lasting results. This includes making room for the occasional treat or indulgence to maintain a positive, balanced relationship with food.

A sample day for an endomorph might look like:

- **Breakfast**: Scrambled eggs with spinach and tomatoes, a slice of whole-grain toast, and avocado slices.
- **Lunch**: Grilled chicken salad with mixed greens, cucumbers, bell peppers, quinoa, and a drizzle of olive oil and balsamic vinegar.
- **Snack**: Greek yogurt with berries and a handful of almonds.
- **Dinner**: Baked salmon with roasted sweet potatoes and steamed broccoli.
- **Optional Evening Snack**: Cottage cheese with sliced cucumber or a small handful of walnuts.

This approach supports balanced blood sugar, reduces cravings, and fuels the body without overloading it with excess calories.

3.3 COMMON FOOD MISTAKES AND HOW TO AVOID THEM

Even with the best intentions, certain dietary habits can work against an endomorph's efforts. Being aware of these common pitfalls can help make better choices and enhance the effectiveness of a nutrition plan.

1. Overloading on Carbs- While carbs provide energy, excessive intake, especially of high-glycemic carbs, can easily lead to fat gain in endomorphs. An emphasis on whole grains and vegetables, rather than sugary or starchy foods, helps balance blood sugar. Opt for whole grains and minimize processed carbs.

2. Ignoring Protein- Some endomorphs may under-consume protein, focusing more on carbs or fats. However, skipping protein can lead to reduced muscle mass, slowing the metabolism. Including a protein source in each meal ensures sustained energy and supports muscle maintenance.

3. Drinking High-Calorie Beverages- Sugary drinks, fruit juices, and even certain coffee drinks can contain a large number of empty calories. These can quickly add up without providing satiety. Choosing water, herbal tea, or black coffee as the primary beverages, and saving sugary drinks for rare occasions, can support healthier weight management.

4. Snacking Without Awareness- Mindless snacking, even on seemingly "healthy" options, can lead to unintended calorie consumption. Practicing mindful eating by pre-portioning snacks or setting times for meals can help prevent this. Foods like nuts are nutritious but calorie-dense, so measuring portions can be beneficial.

5. Skipping Meals or Fasting Excessively- While intermittent fasting may benefit some, skipping meals can lead to low energy and subsequent overeating. For endomorphs, balanced and regular meals may be more effective for steady energy and blood sugar levels.

6. Eating Processed "Health Foods"- Many foods marketed as "healthy" are actually loaded with hidden sugars, refined grains, or unhealthy fats. Protein bars, flavored yogurts, and granola can often be high in added sugars. Reading labels and choosing whole, unprocessed foods over packaged options is usually a smarter choice.

CHAPTER 4

CREATING A SUSTAINABLE EATING PLAN

4.1 CALORIC NEEDS AND DEFICIT CALCULATIONS

Understanding your caloric needs is a fundamental part of building a sustainable eating plan. For endomorphs, who may have a naturally lower basal metabolic rate (BMR) and a tendency to store fat, calculating an appropriate calorie intake is essential for weight management and health.

The first step in determining caloric needs is calculating BMR, which is the number of calories your body needs to perform basic functions at rest, such as breathing, circulating blood, and cell repair. BMR can be calculated using formulas like the Harris-Benedict or Mifflin-St Jeor equation, which consider factors such as age, gender, weight, and height. For example:

Mifflin-St Jeor Equation:

- For men: BMR = (10 × weight in kg) + (6.25 × height in cm) - (5 × age) + 5

- For women: BMR = (10 × weight in kg) + (6.25 × height in cm) - (5 × age) - 161

Once you have your BMR, you can factor in your activity level to find your Total Daily Energy Expenditure (TDEE). TDEE accounts for the calories burned through various levels of physical activity, from sedentary to highly active lifestyles. By multiplying your BMR by the appropriate activity factor, you get an estimate of how many calories you need to maintain your current weight.

To create a calorie deficit for weight loss, endomorphs should aim to consume fewer calories than their TDEE. A common approach is to start with a modest deficit of 15-20% below the TDEE, which is usually sustainable and won't overly tax the body. For example, if your TDEE is 2,000 calories, a 20% deficit would put you at 1,600 calories per day. This amount is generally enough to stimulate weight loss without triggering intense hunger or energy crashes.

However, endomorphs should avoid overly drastic calorie restrictions. Extreme deficits may lead to muscle loss, slow metabolism further, and increase the likelihood of weight regain. It's better to aim for a steady, gradual weight loss rate of around 0.5 to 1 pound per week, which supports long-term sustainability and minimizes the risk of metabolic adaptation (where the body slows down to conserve energy in response to fewer calories).

Regularly reassessing your caloric needs as you progress is also key. As you lose weight, your BMR and TDEE decrease, which means adjusting your intake to avoid plateaus.

4.2 MEAL TIMING AND FREQUENCY FOR OPTIMAL METABOLISM

Meal timing and frequency can play an important role in managing hunger, energy, and metabolism—especially for endomorphs, who may benefit from strategies that stabilize blood sugar levels and reduce insulin spikes. While there isn't a single "best" way to time meals, certain strategies may help endomorphs optimize their eating patterns.

1. Eating Small, Balanced Meals Throughout the Day
Some endomorphs find that consuming 4-6 smaller meals spread throughout the day can help maintain stable blood sugar levels and prevent energy dips. These meals should

ideally include protein, fiber, and healthy fats to promote satiety. This approach can reduce overeating by preventing the extreme hunger that sometimes leads to impulsive food choices.

2. Prioritizing Protein in the Morning- Starting the day with a high-protein breakfast can jump-start the metabolism and reduce cravings later in the day. Protein helps regulate appetite hormones like ghrelin (which triggers hunger) and leptin (which promotes satiety), making it easier to avoid unnecessary snacking. Eggs, Greek yogurt, or a protein-rich smoothie with vegetables can all be effective breakfast options.

3. Avoiding Late-Night Eating- While the effect of late-night eating varies among individuals, endomorphs may benefit from limiting food intake closer to bedtime. Eating large meals late at night can disrupt sleep and may impact insulin sensitivity, leading to more fat storage over time. Aiming to finish meals at least 2-3 hours before bed allows the body to digest and stabilize before sleep.

4. Incorporating Intermittent Fasting (Optional)- Intermittent fasting (IF) has gained popularity for its potential metabolic benefits, including improved insulin sensitivity and easier calorie management. IF typically involves an eating window (e.g., 8 hours) and a fasting period (e.g., 16 hours). While this approach doesn't suit everyone, some endomorphs find it helpful for reducing overall calorie intake and simplifying meal timing. However, it's important to ensure that meals within the eating window are nutrient-dense and balanced to prevent nutrient deficiencies.

5. Timing Carbohydrates Around Activity- For endomorphs who exercise regularly, consuming most carbohydrates around workout times can improve energy levels and muscle recovery. This approach, known as carb timing, provides fuel for workouts and supports post-exercise muscle repair. Consuming complex carbs, like oats or sweet potatoes, an hour or so before a workout can provide sustained energy, while a balanced meal with protein and carbs post-workout can aid recovery.

Ultimately, the key to meal timing is to find a structure that fits individual preferences and lifestyle. Sticking to a consistent meal pattern that supports energy, reduces cravings, and prevents overeating will contribute to a more sustainable eating plan.

4.3 SAMPLE MEAL PLANS AND FOOD LISTS

Crafting a balanced, endomorph-friendly meal plan can help support weight management, muscle retention, and overall wellness. Below are two sample day plans that emphasize balanced macronutrient intake and nutrient-dense, whole foods.

Sample Meal Plan 1

- **Breakfast**:
  - Scrambled eggs (2-3) with spinach and tomatoes, cooked in a small amount of olive oil
  - 1 slice whole-grain toast
  - 1/2 avocado
- **Mid-Morning Snack**:
  - Greek yogurt (unsweetened) with fresh berries and a small handful of almonds
- **Lunch**:
  - Grilled chicken breast over a large salad with mixed greens, cucumbers, bell peppers, and a handful of quinoa

- o Drizzled with olive oil and balsamic vinegar
- **Afternoon Snack**:
- o Veggie sticks (carrot, celery, bell pepper) with hummus
- **Dinner**:
- o Baked salmon with a side of roasted sweet potatoes and steamed broccoli
- o Mixed green side salad with olive oil and lemon juice
- **Evening Snack (Optional)**:
- o Cottage cheese with sliced cucumber or a few cherry tomatoes

---

Sample Meal Plan 2

- **Breakfast**:
- o High-protein smoothie with unsweetened almond milk, a handful of spinach, 1/2 banana, a scoop of protein powder, and a tablespoon of chia seeds
- **Mid-Morning Snack**:
- o Cottage cheese with cucumber slices and a few walnuts
- **Lunch**:
- o Turkey and veggie wrap using a whole-grain tortilla, with mixed greens, sliced peppers, and a light drizzle of mustard or olive oil

- **Afternoon Snack**:
- o Apple slices with almond butter
- **Dinner**:
- o Stir-fried tofu or lean beef with mixed vegetables (like bell peppers, broccoli, and snap peas) over a small serving of brown rice or quinoa
- **Evening Snack (Optional)**:
- o A handful of pumpkin seeds or a small piece of dark chocolate

---

Food List for Endomorph-Friendly Meals

Protein Sources:

- Lean meats (chicken breast, turkey)
- Fish (salmon, tuna)
- Eggs and egg whites
- Greek yogurt (unsweetened)
- Cottage cheese
- Plant-based proteins (tofu, tempeh)
- Legumes (chickpeas, lentils)

Carbohydrates:

- Vegetables (spinach, kale, bell peppers, broccoli, zucchini)
- Low-glycemic fruits (berries, apples, pears)
- Whole grains (quinoa, oats, brown rice, farro)
- Starchy vegetables (sweet potatoes, pumpkin)
- Legumes and beans (black beans, lentils)

Healthy Fats:

- Avocado
- Nuts and seeds (almonds, chia seeds, walnuts, pumpkin seeds)
- Olive oil and coconut oil
- Nut butters (almond, peanut—unsweetened)
- Fatty fish (salmon, sardines)

Fiber-Rich Foods:

- Vegetables (artichokes, Brussels sprouts)
- Fruits (berries, apples, pears)
- Whole grains and oats
- Legumes and beans
- Nuts and seeds

CHAPTER 5

EXERCISE STRATEGIES FOR ENDOMORPHS

5.1 THE ROLE OF CARDIO VS. STRENGTH TRAINING

When it comes to exercise, many people automatically think of cardio as the go-to method for weight loss. However, for endomorphs, the balance between cardio and strength training is crucial for effective and sustainable weight loss.

1. Cardio for Calorie Burn and Fat Loss- Cardiovascular exercises—like running, cycling, and swimming—are effective for burning calories and enhancing cardiovascular health. Since endomorphs have a tendency to store fat, cardio can be a useful tool for burning extra calories and creating the caloric deficit needed for weight loss. However, the type and amount of cardio should be managed carefully to prevent muscle loss and metabolic slowdown, which can be counterproductive.

Best Cardio Options for Endomorphs:

- **Moderate-Intensity Steady-State (MISS) Cardio**: Endomorphs can benefit from moderate-intensity cardio for 30-45 minutes, 3-4 times per week. This could include brisk walking, light jogging, or cycling. MISS helps burn calories without the risk of muscle loss that can come with prolonged high-intensity cardio.

- **High-Intensity Interval Training (HIIT)**: Short bursts of high-intensity cardio, followed by rest or low-intensity periods, can stimulate metabolism and burn more fat in less time. We'll cover HIIT in more detail in the next section, as it's particularly effective for endomorphs.

2. Strength Training for Muscle Building and Metabolic Boost

Strength training is an essential component for endomorphs, as building muscle helps increase the resting metabolic rate (RMR). Muscle is metabolically active, meaning it burns more calories at rest than fat tissue. By increasing muscle mass, endomorphs can improve their metabolism and promote a leaner physique.

Best Strength Training Options for Endomorphs:

- **Compound Movements**: Exercises like squats, deadlifts, bench presses, and rows work multiple muscle groups simultaneously and have a higher calorie burn compared to isolation exercises. Compound movements also stimulate muscle growth and improve overall strength.

- **Full-Body Workouts**: Focusing on full-body strength sessions, rather than isolating individual muscle groups, can help endomorphs maximize calorie burn and prevent muscle imbalances. Aim for 3-4 sessions per week, incorporating all major muscle groups.

- **Moderate Reps with Challenging Weights**: Reps in the range of 8-12 with a weight that's challenging by the final reps is typically effective for building muscle and strength. Avoid excessively high reps or very light weights, as these may not stimulate enough muscle growth.

The combination of cardio and strength training can optimize results, supporting both fat loss and muscle retention. Cardio burns calories, while strength training builds a muscular foundation that contributes to long-term metabolic health.

5.2 HIIT WORKOUTS AND METABOLIC BOOST

High-Intensity Interval Training (HIIT) has become popular for a reason: it's efficient and effective at boosting metabolism and burning fat. HIIT involves short bursts of intense exercise (e.g., sprinting or jumping) followed by rest or low-intensity activity. This method is particularly beneficial for endomorphs because it not only burns calories during the workout but also elevates metabolism for hours afterward through a phenomenon known as the "afterburn effect" or excess post-exercise oxygen consumption (EPOC).

Benefits of HIIT for Endomorphs:

- **Maximized Calorie Burn**: HIIT workouts can burn a high number of calories in a short amount of time. This is particularly helpful for endomorphs who want to create a calorie deficit without spending hours at the gym.
- **Increased Metabolism**: The EPOC effect means that endomorphs continue to burn calories after the workout, contributing to a higher overall calorie burn throughout the day.

- **Preservation of Lean Muscle**: Unlike steady-state cardio, which can sometimes lead to muscle loss when overdone, HIIT tends to be muscle-sparing. The short bursts of intensity help retain muscle mass while focusing on fat burn.

Sample HIIT Workout for Endomorphs: Here's a 20-minute HIIT routine that can be done 2-3 times a week. Warm up first with light cardio (e.g., jogging or jumping jacks) for 5 minutes.

1. **30 seconds of sprinting (or high knees)**
   - Rest for 30 seconds.
2. **30 seconds of burpees**
   - Rest for 30 seconds.
3. **30 seconds of mountain climbers**
   - Rest for 30 seconds.
4. **30 seconds of jumping squats**
   - Rest for 30 seconds.

Repeat this circuit 3-4 times. HIIT sessions don't need to be long to be effective—just 20-30 minutes a few times a week can yield significant results when paired with strength training.

5.3 DESIGNING A WEEKLY WORKOUT ROUTINE

A well-rounded weekly workout plan can help endomorphs achieve their weight loss and muscle-building goals effectively. Here's a sample weekly schedule that balances strength training, cardio, and rest for optimal results:

Weekly Workout Plan for Endomorphs

- **Monday: Strength Training (Full Body)**
  - Focus on compound movements such as squats, deadlifts, push-ups, and rows.
  - Aim for 3 sets of 8-12 reps for each exercise.
- **Tuesday: HIIT Cardio**
  - Perform a 20-30 minute HIIT session, alternating between high-intensity exercises (e.g., sprinting, jump squats) and rest periods.
- **Wednesday: Active Rest or Light Cardio**
  - Opt for a low-intensity activity, such as brisk walking or cycling, for 30-45 minutes.
  - Alternatively, use this day for gentle stretching or yoga to improve flexibility.
- **Thursday: Strength Training (Full Body)**

- Another full-body session, possibly using different exercises or variations from Monday.
- Include exercises like lunges, shoulder presses, kettlebell swings, or planks.

- **Friday: Steady-State Cardio**
- Engage in a moderate-intensity cardio session, such as a 40-minute jog, cycling, or swimming.

- **Saturday: Strength Training and Core Work**
- Incorporate core-focused exercises like planks, Russian twists, or hanging leg raises.
- Continue full-body strength exercises to support muscle growth.

- **Sunday: Rest or Active Recovery**
- Rest is crucial for muscle recovery and preventing overtraining.
- Light stretching, foam rolling, or gentle yoga can promote circulation and reduce soreness.

This schedule combines a variety of exercises to ensure all muscle groups are engaged while avoiding burnout. It provides a good mix of intensity, targeting both fat loss and muscle growth. The strength training sessions promote muscle retention, while the cardio and HIIT sessions help create a calorie deficit and support cardiovascular health.

Key Tips for Exercise Success

1. Start with a Warm-Up and End with a Cool-Down
Each workout should begin with a 5-10 minute warm-up to prepare your body, and end with stretching to improve flexibility and aid in recovery.

2. Track Progress and Adjust as Needed Regularly track your strength, endurance, and body measurements to assess progress. If you're no longer progressing, consider adjusting weights, intensity, or rest periods to continue challenging yourself.

3. Prioritize Consistency Over Intensity While high-intensity workouts are effective, consistency is what drives long-term results. Finding a routine you can stick with is more important than doing extreme workouts that may lead to burnout.

4. Listen to Your Body Endomorphs should avoid overtraining, as this can lead to injuries and slow down progress. Prioritize adequate rest and be mindful of any signs of fatigue or strain.

CHAPTER 6

BOOSTING METABOLISM NATURALLY

6.1 FOODS AND NUTRIENTS THAT INCREASE METABOLIC RATE

The foods we eat impact our metabolism in powerful ways. Certain foods and nutrients can provide a natural boost to the metabolic rate, which is particularly beneficial for endomorphs aiming to overcome a naturally slower metabolism.

1. Protein-Rich Foods- Protein has a high thermic effect of food (TEF), meaning the body expends more energy digesting and metabolizing protein than it does carbohydrates or fats. High-protein foods can temporarily increase metabolism by 15-30%, while carbohydrates and fats increase it by only 5-10% and 0-3%, respectively. Foods rich in protein, such as lean meats, fish, eggs, tofu, legumes, and Greek yogurt, can help endomorphs increase calorie burn during digestion and support muscle growth, which contributes to a higher resting metabolic rate (RMR).

2. Foods High in Fiber- Fiber not only aids digestion but also helps regulate blood sugar levels and increase satiety, which can prevent overeating. High-fiber foods, like whole grains, vegetables, fruits, and legumes, slow down digestion and support healthy gut bacteria, both of which are linked to improved metabolic function. A high-fiber diet also encourages the body to utilize fat stores for energy, aiding in weight loss.

3. Green Tea and Coffee- Green tea and coffee are known for their metabolism-boosting properties, thanks to their caffeine content. Caffeine is a natural stimulant that can temporarily increase energy expenditure and fat oxidation. Green tea also contains catechins, which work synergistically with caffeine to enhance metabolism and fat burning. Consuming 2-3 cups of green tea or coffee daily can support calorie burn, though it's essential to avoid excessive intake, as this can lead to negative side effects like jitteriness or disrupted sleep.

4. Spices Like Cayenne Pepper and Ginger- Certain spices have thermogenic properties, meaning they can temporarily increase body temperature and boost metabolism. Cayenne pepper contains capsaicin, which has been shown to enhance fat burning and decrease appetite.

Similarly, ginger promotes digestion and raises metabolic rate. Incorporating these spices into meals is a simple way to enhance flavor and support metabolism.

5. Omega-3 Fatty Acids- Omega-3 fatty acids, found in fatty fish (such as salmon, mackerel, and sardines), flaxseeds, and chia seeds, can help reduce inflammation and improve metabolic health. Omega-3s have been shown to reduce insulin resistance, which is particularly beneficial for endomorphs who may be prone to metabolic issues. These healthy fats also support muscle retention, which in turn helps maintain a higher metabolic rate.

6. Water-Rich Foods and Adequate Hydration- Staying hydrated is essential for optimal metabolism. Even mild dehydration can slow down the metabolic rate. Water-rich foods, such as cucumbers, watermelon, and lettuce, contribute to hydration, and drinking water throughout the day supports efficient calorie-burning processes. Studies suggest that drinking cold water may increase metabolic rate temporarily, as the body expends energy warming the water to body temperature.

Incorporating these metabolism-boosting foods into a daily diet can support calorie burn, reduce hunger, and make weight loss more manageable for endomorphs.

6.2 LIFESTYLE HABITS TO ACCELERATE FAT BURN

Diet is only one part of the equation. Lifestyle habits play a critical role in maintaining a healthy metabolism and maximizing fat burn.

1. Regular Physical Activity- Staying active throughout the day helps prevent metabolic slowdown and increases calorie burn. For endomorphs, adding "non-exercise activity thermogenesis" (NEAT) activities, like walking, cleaning, or standing, can make a significant difference. Small lifestyle changes, such as taking the stairs instead of the elevator or parking farther from entrances, can add up to increased energy expenditure.

2. Strength Training- Muscle is metabolically active tissue, meaning that the more muscle mass one has, the more calories are burned at rest. Regular strength training helps endomorphs build and retain muscle, boosting resting metabolic rate. Compound exercises like squats, deadlifts, and push-ups are especially effective, as they engage multiple muscle groups and stimulate greater calorie burn.

3. High-Intensity Interval Training (HIIT)- HIIT involves alternating between short, intense bursts of exercise and rest periods, resulting in a significant post-exercise calorie burn. This form of exercise boosts the metabolism through the "afterburn effect" (excess post-exercise oxygen consumption, or EPOC), where the body continues burning calories even after the workout is over. Just two or three 20-30 minute HIIT sessions per week can contribute to faster metabolism and fat loss.

4. Fidgeting and Standing More Often- Surprisingly, even small movements like fidgeting, stretching, and shifting positions can contribute to increased calorie burn. Studies show that people who fidget or move throughout the day can burn up to several hundred more calories than those who remain sedentary. Standing desks or frequent breaks to walk around can help endomorphs stay active and boost their metabolic rate.

5. Keeping a Consistent Meal Schedule- Eating at regular intervals can support a steady metabolism. While intermittent fasting is popular, some endomorphs may find that eating every 3-4 hours helps prevent large insulin spikes and keeps energy levels stable. Consistent meal timing can also prevent intense hunger, which can lead to overeating.

6.3 MANAGING STRESS AND SLEEP FOR OPTIMAL METABOLISM

Stress and poor sleep are often overlooked factors that significantly affect metabolism. Both of these elements influence hormone levels, which can impact hunger, energy, and fat storage.

1. Managing Stress Levels- Chronic stress triggers the release of cortisol, a hormone associated with fat storage, particularly in the abdominal area. High cortisol levels also interfere with insulin regulation, increasing the likelihood of weight gain. Incorporating stress-reducing practices like meditation, deep breathing exercises, yoga, or journaling can help endomorphs manage cortisol levels, thus reducing the risk of stress-induced weight gain.

2. Prioritizing Quality Sleep- Sleep is essential for metabolic health. Poor or insufficient sleep disrupts the balance of hunger hormones, ghrelin, and leptin, making it more likely to experience increased appetite and cravings. Sleep deprivation also affects insulin sensitivity, which can lead to higher fat storage and make it more challenging for endomorphs to lose weight.

Aiming for 7-9 hours of quality sleep each night supports hormone regulation and improves the body's ability to burn calories efficiently. Good sleep hygiene practices include:

- Establishing a consistent sleep schedule
- Limiting caffeine and screen time before bed
- Creating a relaxing bedtime routine to promote restful sleep

3. Limiting Blue Light Exposure- Blue light from screens (like smartphones, computers, and TVs) can interfere with melatonin production, the hormone that regulates sleep. Melatonin not only promotes restful sleep but also influences energy metabolism. Reducing screen time an hour before bed or using blue light filters can support better sleep quality, which ultimately benefits metabolic health.

4. Practicing Mindful Eating- Stress can lead to emotional eating or eating out of habit rather than hunger, which is especially challenging for endomorphs. Practicing mindful eating—focusing on hunger cues, savoring each bite, and eating slowly—can prevent overeating and support a balanced metabolism. Mindful eating helps endomorphs make conscious food choices and avoid the stress-eating pitfalls that can interfere with weight loss goals.

CHAPTER 7

TRACKING PROGRESS AND STAYING MOTIVATED

7.1 SETTING REALISTIC GOALS

A clear, achievable goal serves as a roadmap, guiding your actions and helping you stay focused. For endomorphs, who may have a natural tendency to gain weight more easily, setting realistic and specific goals is especially important.

1. Understanding SMART Goals- SMART goals— Specific, Measurable, Achievable, Relevant, and Time-bound—are a proven method for setting clear, realistic goals. Instead of a vague goal like "lose weight," a SMART goal would be: "I want to lose 10 pounds in three months by following a balanced diet and working out five days a week." This goal is:

- **Specific**: It defines the exact amount of weight to lose.
- **Measurable**: Progress can be tracked in pounds lost.
- **Achievable**: A 10-pound loss over three months is manageable.
- **Relevant**: Weight loss is aligned with the larger health goal.
- **Time-bound**: A three-month timeline adds structure.

2. Focusing on Long-Term Health- For endomorphs, weight loss can be slower, and focusing only on the scale can lead to frustration. Instead, emphasize long-term health benefits, such as improved energy, strength, and metabolic function. Goals like "reduce body fat by 5%," "gain muscle mass," or "improve endurance" can help endomorphs stay motivated even when the scale isn't moving dramatically.

3. Setting Process-Oriented Goals- Process-oriented goals focus on actions rather than outcomes. For instance, instead of only aiming to lose a certain amount of weight, set goals such as "I will meal prep every Sunday," "I will exercise five times a week," or "I will drink eight glasses of water each day." Process goals help build habits and maintain motivation, regardless of how quickly results appear.

4. Celebrating Milestones- Setting small milestones within larger goals keeps motivation high. Celebrating non-scale victories, like increasing weights during strength training, completing a 5K run, or noticing improved sleep quality, reinforces progress and helps endomorphs stay positive throughout their journey.

7.2 HOW TO MEASURE BODY COMPOSITION AND TRACK WEIGHT LOSS

Tracking progress accurately is essential for staying motivated and making adjustments to your fitness plan as needed. While weight is one metric, focusing solely on the scale can be misleading. Other measurements, such as body composition and circumferences, give a more comprehensive view of your progress.

1. Using Body Composition Measurements Body composition measurements provide insight into fat and muscle percentages rather than just overall weight. Endomorphs, who may see slower progress on the scale due to muscle gain, can benefit from tracking body fat percentage. Several methods are available:

- **Body Fat Calipers**: Calipers measure skinfold thickness at various body sites. While they require some practice to use accurately, they're a cost-effective option.

- **Bioelectrical Impedance Scales**: These scales send a weak electrical current through the body to estimate body fat. While not as accurate as other methods, they offer an easy and consistent way to track trends over time.

- **DEXA Scans or Body Composition Analysis**: These are more precise but often costly and may require a visit to a clinic or fitness center.

2.   Tracking   Weight   and   Circumference
While body weight isn't the only indicator of progress, regular weigh-ins can be useful if interpreted correctly. Weigh yourself once a week, ideally under similar conditions each time (e.g., same time of day, same clothing). In addition to weighing yourself, take circumference measurements around key areas like the waist, hips, thighs, and arms. Tracking inches lost can be

more encouraging than focusing solely on pounds, as it reflects both fat loss and muscle gain.

3.   Monitoring   Fitness   and   Performance Physical progress isn't just about fat loss. Tracking improvements in fitness, like increased strength, stamina, and flexibility, can show that you're making progress even if the scale doesn't move. Record the weights you lift, reps and sets completed, or times for running distances. These are tangible indicators of your growing strength and endurance.

4.   Using   Photos   and   Journals Progress photos can reveal physical changes that may not show up on the scale. Take photos once a month, wearing similar clothing and under similar lighting. Additionally, consider keeping a fitness journal to log meals, workouts, and thoughts. A journal can help you identify patterns, track moods, and note any factors affecting progress.

7.3 TIPS FOR STAYING MOTIVATED AND OVERCOMING PLATEAUS

Maintaining motivation over the long term, especially when progress slows down, is essential for reaching your weight loss goals. Endomorphs may encounter plateaus, but by adjusting your mindset and strategies, you can overcome these challenges.

1. Embracing a Growth Mindset- A growth mindset means viewing setbacks as opportunities to learn rather than as failures. Plateaus or slow progress should be seen as a natural part of the journey, prompting you to reevaluate and adjust rather than give up. For instance, if weight loss stalls, it might be time to tweak your diet, increase workout intensity, or vary your routine.

2. Mixing Up Workouts- Endomorphs may experience plateaus if they repeat the same workouts over and over. The body becomes efficient at familiar routines, and calorie burn may decrease. To break through a plateau, try varying exercises, adding HIIT sessions, increasing weights in strength training, or exploring a new fitness class. These changes not only keep workouts interesting but also challenge muscles in new ways.

3. Surrounding Yourself with Support- Having a support system can make a huge difference in staying motivated. Friends, family, or a workout buddy can encourage and help hold you accountable. Alternatively, consider joining a fitness group or online community where others are working toward similar goals. Sharing progress and challenges can boost motivation and provide new ideas for overcoming obstacles.

4. Practicing Self-Compassion- Weight loss journeys often come with emotional highs and lows. Practicing self-compassion means acknowledging your efforts and treating yourself kindly, even when progress slows. Endomorphs, who may face more challenges in losing weight, can benefit from focusing on the positive changes they're making rather than on any perceived shortcomings.

5. Reassessing Your Goals- If you've reached a plateau, it may be worth revisiting your goals. Perhaps your initial goal was to lose a specific amount of weight, but you've since developed a love for strength training. Adjusting your goals to reflect new interests, like building muscle or improving endurance, can help reignite motivation. Sometimes, a shift in focus brings renewed excitement to your fitness journey.

6. Visualizing Success and Using Positive Affirmations
Visualization and affirmations can be powerful motivators.
Spend a few minutes each day visualizing yourself reaching
your goals, whether that's feeling confident, lifting heavier
weights, or running a race. Positive affirmations like "I am
committed to my health and fitness" or "Every step I take is
bringing me closer to my goal" can reinforce your resolve.

7. Rewarding Yourself Along the Way- Celebrate your
hard work with non-food rewards when you hit milestones.
Treat yourself to new workout gear, a relaxing massage, or
a weekend getaway. Rewards create positive associations
with progress and provide extra motivation to keep pushing
forward.

CHAPTER 8

DEALING WITH COMMON SETBACKS

8.1 UNDERSTANDING WEIGHT LOSS PLATEAUS

A weight loss plateau happens when progress seems to
stall, even when you're maintaining your routine. For
endomorphs, whose bodies are naturally inclined to store

fat, plateaus can be frustrating but are also a normal part of the weight loss process.

1. Why Plateaus Happen- Plateaus occur because as you lose weight, your body requires fewer calories to function. When you begin a diet and exercise plan, the initial weight loss often includes a mix of fat, water, and even muscle loss. But as your body adapts, it becomes more efficient, and the calorie deficit you created at the start is no longer enough to prompt further loss. This adaptive response is part of your body's effort to maintain balance, or homeostasis.

2. The Importance of Tracking Adjustments- One effective way to address plateaus is by recalibrating your caloric intake and exercise intensity. Start by reassessing your caloric needs, as they may have changed since the beginning of your journey. Reducing your daily intake by 100–200 calories or increasing your physical activity slightly can help restart weight loss. Strength training is particularly helpful for endomorphs, as building muscle can increase your resting metabolic rate and counteract the metabolic slowdown that contributes to plateaus.

3. Focusing on Non-Scale Victories- Sometimes, weight loss isn't visible on the scale, but you may still be making progress in other ways. Improved stamina, better mood, greater flexibility, or even fitting into clothes differently are all indicators of success. Focusing on these non-scale victories helps you maintain a positive perspective and motivates you to continue pushing through.

4. Periodically Changing Your Routine- The body can become accustomed to repetitive exercise routines, so regularly changing things up is beneficial. For example, if you usually do steady-state cardio, try incorporating high-intensity interval training (HIIT). If your workout relies heavily on cardio, adding strength training can revamp your approach. Variations challenge your muscles in new ways and help avoid boredom, making your workouts more engaging and effective.

8.2 HOW TO AVOID BURNOUT AND STAY CONSISTENT

Burnout can be a major obstacle to progress, especially when combined with the natural challenges of weight loss for endomorphs. Staying consistent requires a mix of motivation, realistic goal-setting, and self-compassion.

1. Setting Sustainable Goals- Setting realistic, achievable goals can keep you from feeling overwhelmed. Many people experience burnout because they set overly ambitious targets, such as trying to lose weight too quickly or exercising every single day without rest. Instead, aim for manageable changes that fit into your life and allow for flexibility, such as setting a goal of working out four times per week or losing one pound per week.

2. Building in Rest and Recovery- Rest days are essential to recovery, particularly for endomorphs whose muscles may need a bit more recovery time due to intense strength training. Without proper rest, you risk overtraining, which can lead to exhaustion and even injury. Design your fitness schedule to include at least one or two rest days each week, and remember that rest days can still include gentle activities like stretching or yoga, which support both body and mind.

3. Avoiding Perfectionism- Perfectionism often leads to an all-or-nothing mindset, which can derail progress. Instead of expecting yourself to follow your diet and exercise plan perfectly, allow room for flexibility and imperfections. If you miss a workout or have an unplanned treat, acknowledge it, learn from it, and move on. Embrace the idea of progress over perfection, which will help you stay consistent over time.

4. Finding Enjoyment in the Process- When you view exercise and healthy eating as chores, burnout is more likely. Look for ways to make your routine enjoyable by choosing activities you genuinely like, whether that's dancing, swimming, or hiking. Experiment with new recipes, explore different forms of exercise, and treat your journey as an opportunity for growth rather than a temporary struggle. Enjoyment breeds consistency, making you more likely to stick with your habits in the long run.

5. Focusing on Self-Care Beyond Weight Loss- Mental and emotional self-care is equally important in staying motivated. Burnout often arises when weight loss becomes the sole focus, creating pressure and frustration. Schedule regular self-care activities that help you relax and recharge, such as meditation, reading, or spending time with friends. A balanced lifestyle is more sustainable and leads to better overall well-being.

8.3 MANAGING SOCIAL SITUATIONS AND FOOD TEMPTATIONS

Social situations can present unique challenges, especially when it comes to food. Navigating parties, holidays, and gatherings without derailing progress requires planning and flexibility.

1. Planning Ahead- One of the best ways to handle social events is to plan in advance. If you're going to a party or dinner, eat a light but protein-rich snack beforehand to curb hunger and make it easier to resist overeating. Research the menu if you're going to a restaurant, and choose options that align with your goals. Planning doesn't mean you have to deprive yourself but rather helps you make conscious choices.

2. Practicing Portion Control- If you want to enjoy a particular food, try focusing on portion control rather than complete restriction. For instance, if you're craving dessert, opt for a smaller portion to satisfy your craving without going overboard. Similarly, when at a buffet or party, start with a small plate and choose a few items you genuinely want to enjoy.

3. Setting Boundaries and Communicating Your Goals
Well-meaning friends or family members might encourage you to indulge, which can make staying on track difficult. Politely communicating your health goals can prevent unwanted pressure. You might say, "I'm working toward my fitness goals, so I'm being mindful of what I eat, but thank you for offering." Setting boundaries helps you stay true to your goals without feeling guilty.

4. Practicing Mindful Eating- Mindful eating is especially helpful in social settings, where it's easy to eat out of habit or social pressure rather than hunger. Take time to savor each bite, pay attention to how you feel, and stop eating when you're satisfied. Mindful eating helps you enjoy food fully and prevents overeating, which can be a common setback in social situations.

5. Allowing Room for Enjoyment- It's important to give yourself permission to enjoy the occasional treat without guilt. Healthy eating is about balance, not deprivation. If you have a meal or snack that doesn't align with your regular routine, let yourself enjoy it fully, then return to your normal plan at the next meal. Flexibility fosters a healthy relationship with food, which is essential for long-term success.

CHAPTER 9

MINDFULNESS AND MENTAL HEALTH IN WEIGHT LOSS

9.1 THE PSYCHOLOGY OF EATING AND SELF-CONTROL

The psychology of eating and self-control is complex, shaped by a variety of factors including emotions, environment, habits, and biological responses. Understanding why we eat, as well as the psychological triggers behind eating behaviors, can empower endomorphs to make more mindful choices.

1. Emotional Eating and Its Triggers- For many people, food serves as a source of comfort during times of stress, sadness, or boredom. This is known as emotional eating, where food is used as a coping mechanism rather than to satisfy hunger. For endomorphs, emotional eating can be particularly challenging, as their body type may store fat more easily, leading to greater weight gain when indulging in high-calorie comfort foods.

Identifying emotional triggers is a critical first step. Triggers can include stress from work, relationship issues, or even celebratory events. By recognizing the specific situations that lead to emotional eating, it becomes easier to find alternative coping mechanisms. Activities like walking, talking to a friend, or practicing deep breathing exercises can serve as healthy replacements for eating when emotions are high.

2. The Role of Dopamine and Reward Mechanisms- Eating releases dopamine, a feel-good neurotransmitter that activates the brain's reward center. Foods high in sugar, salt, and fat are especially potent in triggering dopamine responses, which can lead to cravings and, over time, reinforce a habit of reaching for such foods in stressful situations. Recognizing this response can help in developing strategies to reduce dependency on high-calorie comfort foods and instead seek pleasure in healthier sources, like physical activity or creative hobbies.

3. Building Self-Control Through Mindfulness- Self-control in eating is a skill that can be cultivated through mindfulness. By practicing mindfulness, you train yourself to slow down, pay attention to the present moment, and observe your eating impulses without immediately acting on them. This awareness allows you to notice the difference between physical hunger and emotional cravings, which is crucial for developing self-control.

Self-control doesn't mean total deprivation; instead, it's about consciously choosing when and what to eat based on physical needs rather than emotional impulses. Learning to pause before eating, assessing hunger levels, and setting intentions for each meal can help you gradually build a habit of self-regulated eating.

9.2 BUILDING A POSITIVE RELATIONSHIP WITH FOOD

A healthy relationship with food is essential for sustainable weight loss and mental well-being. Food is often tied to cultural, social, and emotional experiences, and it's easy to fall into patterns of guilt, shame, or restriction, especially in a weight-loss journey. Building a positive relationship with food allows endomorphs to enjoy a balanced diet without stress or guilt.

1. Letting Go of Food Labels- One way to improve your relationship with food is to stop categorizing foods as "good" or "bad." While some foods are more nutrient-dense than others, labeling foods can create feelings of guilt when eating certain items and can contribute to a cycle of restriction and overeating. By viewing food neutrally, you'll find it easier to make balanced choices without falling into the "all-or-nothing" mindset. Instead of focusing on restriction, aim for moderation and include a variety of foods that provide both nourishment and enjoyment.

2. Practicing Self-Compassion Around Food Choices
Self-compassion involves treating yourself with kindness,

even when you make mistakes. For endomorphs, weight loss can be a slower process, and it's easy to feel discouraged by setbacks. Practicing self-compassion around food choices means forgiving yourself if you overeat or indulge, rather than falling into a spiral of guilt. Remind yourself that one meal or snack doesn't define your progress and that every day is an opportunity to make a choice that aligns with your goals.

3. Fostering Gratitude for Food and Nourishment
Fostering a sense of gratitude toward food can shift your perspective from focusing solely on calories and weight loss to appreciating food for its ability to nourish your body. Take a moment before each meal to express gratitude for the food on your plate and the nutrients it provides. This simple practice can promote a healthier, more appreciative relationship with eating.

9.3 MINDFUL EATING TECHNIQUES

Mindful eating is a practice that encourages being fully present during meals, paying attention to the sensory experience of food, and making conscious choices. For endomorphs, who may find it easier to gain weight, mindful eating can be an effective tool for portion control, reducing overeating, and cultivating a healthier attitude toward food.

1. Eating Slowly and Savoring Each Bite- One of the simplest yet most powerful mindful eating techniques is to slow down. Eating quickly can lead to overconsumption because it takes about 20 minutes for the brain to register fullness. By eating slowly and taking small bites, you give your body time to signal when it's full, making it easier to avoid overeating. Additionally, savoring each bite allows you to fully enjoy the flavors, textures, and aromas of your food, which can enhance satisfaction.

2. Tuning Into Hunger and Fullness Cues- Before each meal or snack, pause to assess your hunger level. On a scale from 1 to 10, with 1 being extremely hungry and 10 being completely full, try to eat when you're at a moderate level of hunger (around 3 or 4) and stop when you feel comfortably satisfied (around 7). This practice helps you become more in tune with your body's natural hunger and fullness signals, reducing the likelihood of eating out of habit or emotion.

3. Eliminating Distractions During Meals- When eating while distracted—such as watching TV, working, or scrolling through your phone—you're less likely to notice when you're full. To practice mindful eating, eliminate distractions and focus solely on the act of eating. Pay attention to each bite, chew slowly, and take breaks between bites. Eating in a calm, distraction-free environment allows you to be more aware of your food choices and portion sizes.

4. Using the "HALT" Method- The HALT method stands for Hungry, Angry, Lonely, or Tired. Before eating, ask yourself if you're truly hungry or if you're reaching for food due to one of these other emotional states. By identifying the root cause, you can address emotions in ways other than eating. For example, if you're lonely, reaching out to a friend might be more fulfilling than a snack. Using HALT encourages self-awareness and promotes healthier responses to emotions.

5. Practicing Portion Control with Visual Cues Mindful eating can be supported by visual portion control techniques. Using smaller plates, bowls, or utensils can help create the perception of a fuller plate while keeping portions in check. Studies have shown that people tend to eat more when served on larger plates, so downsizing your dinnerware is a simple way to manage portions without feeling deprived.

6. Reflecting After Each Meal- After eating, take a few moments to reflect on the experience. Consider how the meal made you feel physically and emotionally, and whether it satisfied your hunger. This reflection can help you identify patterns and make adjustments. For instance, if a meal left you unsatisfied, you might need to incorporate more protein or fiber next time. Reflection promotes greater awareness of how different foods affect your body and mind.

CHAPTER 10

MAINTAINING WEIGHT LOSS LONG-TERM

10.1 TRANSITIONING TO MAINTENANCE MODE

Once you've successfully reached your weight loss goal, it's important to transition into maintenance mode to prevent regaining the weight. This shift requires you to adjust your approach to eating, exercise, and self-care, while still prioritizing your health and well-being.

1. Gradually Increasing Caloric Intake- One of the most common mistakes people make after losing weight is dramatically increasing their caloric intake, assuming that they can return to pre-weight loss eating habits. However, transitioning too quickly to a higher calorie intake can lead to weight regain, as your body has become accustomed to a lower caloric intake during the weight loss phase.

To transition safely, aim to gradually increase your daily caloric intake by 100 to 200 calories per week. Monitor your weight and adjust accordingly. If you notice the scale creeping upward, reduce your caloric intake slightly. This gradual increase helps your body adjust without overwhelming your metabolism.

2. Adjusting Your Exercise Routine- During weight loss, you may have been focusing heavily on creating a caloric deficit through exercise. In maintenance mode, it's important to continue exercising regularly, but you can reduce the intensity or frequency of your workouts to prevent overtraining and burnout. However, consistency is key. Aim to maintain at least 150 minutes of moderate exercise each week, including a balance of cardio and strength training. Strength training is especially beneficial for endomorphs, as it builds lean muscle, which helps support a healthy metabolism.

3. Monitoring and Tracking- Even in maintenance mode, regular monitoring is essential. Track your weight, body composition, and other relevant health markers periodically to ensure that you are staying on track. It's important to note that your weight may fluctuate slightly, but regular tracking will help you identify trends and make adjustments before small gains turn into larger ones. However, avoid obsessing over the scale—your overall health, fitness, and how your clothes fit are better indicators of success.

10.2 STRATEGIES TO KEEP THE WEIGHT OFF

Maintaining weight loss over the long term isn't just about maintaining a certain number on the scale; it's about adopting strategies that support a sustainable lifestyle. It requires ongoing commitment to healthy habits and an understanding that the process is dynamic.

1. Embrace Flexibility, Not Perfection- One of the keys to long-term maintenance is to adopt a flexible approach to your diet and lifestyle. Perfectionism can create feelings of guilt when you stray from your eating plan, which can trigger unhealthy behaviors. Instead, aim for consistency, not perfection. Allow room for occasional indulgences, like a celebratory dinner or a piece of cake at a birthday party, without viewing these moments as "failures." A healthy relationship with food means knowing how to enjoy treats in moderation without derailing progress.

2. Prioritize Consistent Physical Activity- Staying active is essential for maintaining weight loss, as physical activity helps to regulate metabolism and maintain muscle mass. Incorporate a mix of aerobic exercises, strength training, and flexibility exercises into your routine. Activities like walking, cycling, swimming, or yoga can be enjoyable and low-impact, making them easy to stick with for the long haul. Try to find forms of exercise that you enjoy, as this will make it easier to stay consistent over time.

For endomorphs, strength training is especially important, as it helps to build lean muscle, which increases resting metabolic rate and prevents the accumulation of body fat. Aim for strength training exercises at least two to three times per week to maintain muscle tone and support overall fat loss.

3. Focus on Mindful Eating- Mindful eating, which involves being present and fully engaged during meals, can help you stay connected to your hunger cues and prevent overeating. It also promotes a healthy relationship with food, allowing you to enjoy eating without guilt or stress. Continue practicing mindful eating habits even after reaching your goal weight. This means paying attention to hunger signals, savoring your food, and eating slowly. Mindful eating can help you maintain your weight by preventing unconscious snacking or emotional eating.

4. Continue Tracking Your Progress- While you may not need to track every meal or workout once you're in maintenance mode, periodic check-ins are important. Track your weight, measurements, and how your clothes fit regularly, and assess your energy levels, sleep quality, and overall well-being. Tracking allows you to spot any patterns or changes early on, helping you make adjustments before you regain weight. Regular self-monitoring promotes self-awareness and accountability, which is crucial for long-term success.

5. Build a Support System- Having a strong support system can make all the difference when it comes to maintaining weight loss. Surround yourself with people who encourage your healthy lifestyle, whether that's friends, family, or a weight loss group. Accountability partners can help you stay on track, celebrate your successes, and provide motivation when you feel like giving up. Additionally, support can come from online communities or fitness apps, where you can connect with others who share similar goals.

10.3 BUILDING LASTING HEALTHY HABITS

Sustaining weight loss is not about following a restrictive diet or an unsustainable routine. It's about developing habits that become a natural part of your daily life and align with your long-term health and fitness goals. Here's how you can build lasting healthy habits that support weight maintenance.

1. Set Long-Term Goals- While your initial weight loss goal may be a specific number on the scale, it's important to set long-term health goals that go beyond appearance. Focus on maintaining your strength, flexibility, energy levels, and overall well-being. Setting goals like "increase my strength training reps," "run a 5k," or "maintain my body composition for six months" can help you stay motivated and committed to your health. These goals should be process-focused and sustainable, rather than outcome-based.

2. Create a Routine That Works for You- The most successful weight loss maintainers have established routines that support their healthy lifestyle. Whether it's meal prepping on Sundays, exercising first thing in the morning, or scheduling regular check-ins with a nutritionist, a well-established routine makes healthy choices easier. Routines help prevent decision fatigue and allow you to stay consistent in the long term. Experiment with different habits and create a daily or weekly routine that suits your lifestyle.

3. Practice Self-Compassion and Flexibility- No one is perfect, and maintaining weight loss doesn't mean sticking rigidly to a set plan every day. Life happens—vacations, family celebrations, and stressful work situations can cause temporary disruptions. It's important to practice self-compassion during these times. Instead of getting discouraged or abandoning your efforts, remind yourself that health is a lifelong journey. A flexible attitude allows you to bounce back from setbacks and maintain balance.

4. Invest in Mental and Emotional Well-Being- Physical health and mental well-being go hand in hand. Stress, anxiety, and poor sleep can contribute to overeating or poor food choices, making it harder to maintain weight loss. Invest in practices that promote mental health, such as meditation, journaling, or therapy. By taking care of your emotional needs, you're better equipped to make healthier choices and maintain your weight loss in a balanced and sustainable way.

5. Keep Evolving and Learning- Maintaining weight loss is an ongoing process of learning and growth. Stay curious and open to new information about nutrition, exercise, and self-care. By continually seeking out knowledge and adapting your habits, you ensure that your lifestyle remains aligned with your long-term goals. This mindset helps you stay flexible, so you can adapt to changes in your life and continue thriving.

CHAPTER 11

CONCLUSION

Embarking on a weight loss journey as an endomorph is a unique challenge, but it is also an opportunity for transformation, self-discovery, and empowerment. As you've learned throughout this blueprint, understanding your body type, focusing on nutrition, exercise, and metabolic strategies, and fostering a positive mindset are all essential components of achieving and maintaining weight loss. This final chapter emphasizes the importance of embracing the endomorph journey and moving forward with confidence and positivity, knowing that your efforts will create lasting, meaningful change in your life.

11.1 EMBRACING THE ENDOMORPH JOURNEY

As an endomorph, your body is naturally inclined to store fat, which can make weight loss seem like a tougher, longer road compared to other body types. However, understanding the science behind your metabolism and how to work with your body rather than against it is empowering. The journey of transforming your health and body composition is not about perfection but about consistency, resilience, and learning how to adapt.

1. Accepting Your Body's Unique Characteristics One of the first steps toward success in your weight loss journey is accepting and understanding your body's unique characteristics. Endomorphs tend to have a rounder or softer physique, a naturally slower metabolism, and a tendency to gain weight more easily. However, these traits do not define you. Instead, they serve as a framework for tailoring strategies that work for you, whether that's adjusting your calorie intake, optimizing your workout routine, or focusing on nutrient-dense foods. When you accept your body's natural tendencies, you stop fighting against it and begin working in harmony with it to achieve your goals.

2. Focusing on Long-Term Health, Not Just Weight
Throughout this blueprint, we've emphasized that weight loss isn't only about shedding pounds—it's about fostering a healthier, more balanced lifestyle. For endomorphs, a major challenge in the weight loss process can be the potential for slow progress. But rather than fixating on the number on the scale, it's important to focus on the bigger picture: improving your energy levels, building strength, boosting metabolism, and enhancing your overall health. The more you focus on your health rather than the weight itself, the more rewarding the journey becomes.

3. Developing Self-Compassion- Embarking on a weight loss journey often comes with periods of struggle, setbacks, or moments where progress may feel slow. This is particularly true for endomorphs, whose metabolism may require more time and patience to show visible results. It's important to develop self-compassion during these challenging times. Acknowledge your efforts, celebrate small victories, and don't let occasional setbacks derail your overall commitment. Self-compassion allows you to view each challenge as an opportunity to learn, rather than a failure. This shift in mindset fosters resilience, which is key to long-term success.

4. Celebrating Progress, Not Perfection- Endomorphs often experience gradual progress, and it's easy to become discouraged by the time it takes to reach your desired goals. However, it's essential to remember that lasting changes take time. Celebrate the small victories along the way—whether it's a new personal best in your workouts, a healthier relationship with food, or feeling more energized. Weight loss is not an all-or-nothing endeavor. Progress is progress, and even the smallest positive change is worth recognizing and celebrating. Building these small successes helps to reinforce your commitment and motivates you to continue forward.

11.2 MOVING FORWARD WITH CONFIDENCE AND POSITIVITY

As you move forward on your weight loss journey, the most powerful tool you have is your mindset. Confidence and positivity are crucial not only for reaching your goals but also for maintaining a healthy and sustainable lifestyle over the long term. Shifting your focus from external results to internal growth and well-being will help you stay motivated and on track, even when faced with obstacles.

1. Cultivating a Growth Mindset- The way you approach challenges can significantly impact your success. A growth mindset—believing that you can improve and grow through effort, learning, and perseverance—can transform the way you view your journey. Instead of seeing setbacks as failures, you'll learn to view them as stepping stones toward success. A growth mindset encourages curiosity and a willingness to adapt your approach, allowing you to embrace new ways of eating, exercising, and living that align with your health goals. Keep an open mind, stay patient, and trust in the process.

2. Creating a Vision for Your Future- As you work toward maintaining your weight loss and improving your health, it can be helpful to visualize your future self—your healthier, more confident, and empowered self. Creating a vision of the person you want to become gives you a sense of direction and purpose. Whether it's visualizing yourself fitting into your favorite clothes, running a race, or simply feeling more confident in your body, having a clear vision helps you stay motivated. This mental picture of your future self acts as a reminder of why you started this journey and serves as fuel during times of doubt.

3. Finding Joy in the Process- When you approach weight loss with a sense of joy and excitement, rather than pressure or negativity, the process becomes much more sustainable. For endomorphs, finding a fitness routine that you enjoy—whether it's yoga, strength training, cycling, or dancing—will make staying active feel less like a chore and more like a celebration of what your body can do. The same goes for food. When you focus on the joy of nourishing your body with wholesome, delicious meals, eating becomes an act of self-care rather than restriction or deprivation. Embrace the process, and remember that true transformation is about becoming the best version of yourself, inside and out.

4. Building Resilience in the Face of Challenges- Life is full of unexpected challenges, and your weight loss journey will undoubtedly have its share of ups and downs. Building resilience is essential for overcoming obstacles and staying on track. Resilience involves bouncing back from setbacks, learning from mistakes, and continuing to move forward with determination. For endomorphs, maintaining weight loss may be a lifelong commitment to staying active, eating mindfully, and taking care of your body. By focusing on building mental strength and resilience, you'll be better equipped to handle the bumps along the way and keep making progress.

5. Empowering Yourself Through Knowledge- The more you educate yourself about your body, metabolism, nutrition, and exercise, the more empowered you'll feel in your weight loss journey. As an endomorph, understanding how your body responds to different foods and workout strategies is critical for achieving your goals. Embrace the learning process and make it a priority to stay informed about new approaches to health and fitness. This knowledge gives you the power to make decisions that are right for you and your unique body, making you an active participant in your own transformation.

6. Surrounding Yourself with Positivity- Your environment plays a significant role in shaping your mindset and success. Surround yourself with people who uplift you and support your health goals. Whether it's friends, family, or a community of like-minded individuals, having a support system that encourages you through challenges and celebrates your successes can make a big difference. Positivity is contagious, and being around others who are focused on their health can inspire you to stay motivated and move forward with confidence.

Your journey as an endomorph is unique, and while the road may at times feel challenging, it is also incredibly rewarding. Embrace the process of transformation, celebrate your small wins, and stay patient with yourself. The foundation you've built throughout this blueprint will help you navigate the ups and downs of your journey with confidence and positivity. By focusing on long-term health, building resilience, and fostering a positive mindset, you can maintain your weight loss and live a vibrant, fulfilling life. Moving forward with the tools and knowledge you've gained, you're now equipped to continue your journey toward a healthier, stronger, and more confident you.

www.ingramcontent.com/pod-product-compliance
Lightning Source LLC
Chambersburg PA
CBHW050817250726
48653CB00006B/2268